Ketogenic C[ookbook]

Best Low-Carb & Hig[h-Fat Recipes] for your Everyday Ketogenic Diet

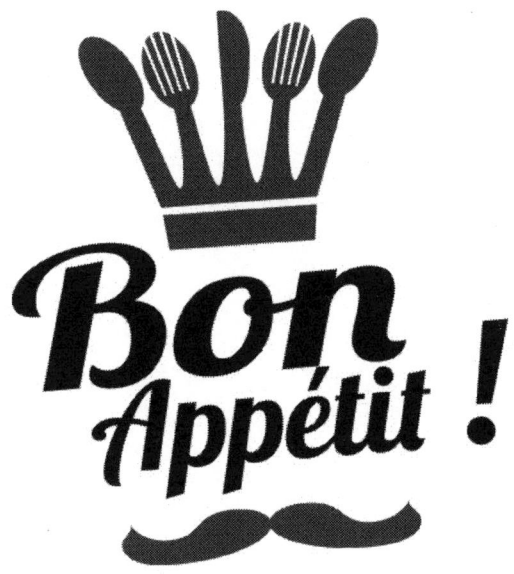

Anthony Evans

Copyright 2017 by Anthony Evans - All rights reserved.

No part of this publication may be reproduced or transmitted in any form or by any means, mechanical or electronic, including photocopying and recording, or by any information storage and retrieval system, without permission, in written, from the author.

All attempts have been made to verify information provided in this publication. Neither the author nor the publisher assumes any responsibility for errors or omissions of the subject matter herein. This publication is not intended for use as a source of legal or accounting advice. The Publisher wants to stress that the information contained herein may be subject to varying state and/or local laws or regulations. All users are advised to retain competent counsel to determine what state and/or local laws or regulations may apply to the user's particular business.

The purchaser or reader of this publication assumes responsibility for the use of these materials and information. Adherence to all applicable laws and regulations, federal, state, and local, governing professional licensing, business practices, advertising, and all other aspects of doing business in the United States or any other jurisdiction is the sole responsibility of the purchaser or reader.

The author and Publisher assume no responsibility or liability whatsoever on the behalf of any purchaser or reader of these materials for injury due to use of any of the methods contained herein. Any perceived slights of specific people or organizations are unintentional.

Contents

CONTENTS 3
INTRODUCTION 7
    What is Ketogenic Diet 7
    Importance of Ketogenic Diet 7
    What to Eat and What to Avoid on Ketogenic Diet? 8
COOKING CONVERSION CHART 13
8 WEIGHT LOSS TIPS 14
BREAKFAST RECIPES 15
    RECIPE 1: CRUSTED TURKEY POTS 15
        Ingredients 15
        Preparation Method 16
        Nutritional Information 16
    RECIPE 2: CABBAGE BREAD 17
        Ingredients 17
        Preparation Method 18
        Nutritional Information 18
    RECIPE 3: FLAX PANCAKES 19
        Ingredients 19
        Preparation Method 19
        Nutritional Information 20
    RECIPE 4: CRUMBLED TURNIP EGGS CUPS 21
        Ingredients 21
        Preparation Method 21
        Nutritional Information 22
LUNCH RECIPES 23
    RECIPE 5: COCONUT PORK STEW 23
        Ingredients 23
        Preparation Method 23
        Nutritional Information 24

RECIPE 6: COCONUT TURKEY STEW..25
   Ingredients 25
   Preparation Method 25
   Nutritional Information..26
RECIPE 7: TURKEY QUICHE 27
   Ingredients 27
   Preparation Method 27
   Nutritional Information..28
RECIPE 8: CABBAGE CHEESE MEAL 29
   Ingredients 29
   Preparation Method 30
   Nutritional Information..30

DINNER RECIPES..31

RECIPE 9: MASCARPONE SALMON WRAPS..............................31
   Ingredients 31
   Preparation Method 31
   Nutritional Information..32
RECIPE 10: VINAIGRETTE LAMB FRY 33
   Ingredients 33
   Preparation Method 33
   Nutritional Information..34
RECIPE 11: GHEE RIND BALLS..35
   Ingredients 35
   Preparation Method 36
   Nutritional Information..36
RECIPE 12: FOREST MUSHROOM BROCCOLI BOWL 37
   Ingredients 37
   Preparation Method 37
   Nutritional Information..38

SOUP RECIPES 39

RECIPE 13: BACON BROCCOLI SOUP.......................................39
   Ingredients 39
   Preparation Method 40
   Nutritional Information..40
RECIPE 14: SOY LAMB SOUP 41
   Ingredients 41

  Preparation Method *41*
  Nutritional Information *42*
 Recipe 15: Lamb Sausage Soup 43
  Ingredients *43*
  Preparation Method *43*
  Nutritional Information *44*
 Recipe 16: Red Chard Cheese Soup 45
  Ingredients *45*
  Preparation Method *45*
  Nutritional Information *46*

SALAD RECIPES 47

 Recipe 17: Sweet Cheese Duck Salad 47
  Ingredients *47*
  Preparation Method *47*
  Nutritional Information *48*
 Recipe 18: Green Nut Salad 49
  Ingredients *49*
  Preparation Method *49*
  Nutritional Information *50*
 Recipe 19: Cheesy Asparagus Salad 51
  Ingredients *51*
  Preparation Method *51*
  Nutritional Information *51*
 Recipe 20: Crab Carrot Salad 53
  Ingredients *53*
  Preparation Method *53*
  Nutritional Information *53*
 Recipe 21: Turkey Salad 55
  Ingredients *55*
  Preparation Method *55*
  Nutritional Information *56*

SNACK RECIPES 57

 Recipe 22: Cabbage Biscuits 57
  Ingredients *57*
  Preparation Method *57*
  Nutritional Information *58*

- Recipe 23: Banana Bombs 59
  - *Ingredients 59*
  - *Preparation Method 59*
  - *Nutritional Information 59*
- Recipe 24: Crunchy Chia Biscuits 61
  - *Ingredients 61*
  - *Preparation Method 61*
  - *Nutritional Information 62*
- Recipe 25: Protein Flax Bars 63
  - *Ingredients 63*
  - *Preparation Method 63*
  - *Nutritional Information 64*
- **CONCLUSION** **65**

Introduction

Thank you for downloading my book **Ketogenic Cookbook: Best Low-Carb & High-Fat Recipes for your Everyday Ketogenic Diet**. I want to believe that this book will help you better understand principles of ketogenic diet and will provide you answers to mostly all your questions.

What is Ketogenic Diet

The ketogenic diet has become very popular nowadays. Its principle is based on the minimum carbohydrates intake and a large fat intake per day. Thanks to this diet your body will constantly be in the stage of ketosis. This is a natural process when the body digests food much more slowly than it usually does. A similar state of the body experiences in the survival mode. In other words, a ketogenic diet is low-carb, high-fat and moderete protein intake which causes the body to burn its own fat to generate energy for everyday life. When you're in the ketogenic diet maximum limit of carbohydrates is not more than 50 grams per day.

Importance of Ketogenic Diet

Ketogenic diet this is not just another trend, it is an effective dieting and for many of us it's a way of life! Its effectiveness is proved not only by weight watchers, but also by those who looking for alternative way of cancer treatment. Maybe it sounds not convincing however, let's consider what ketosis really is.

The process of ketosis in a ketogenic diet is looks like this: glucose supplies every cell of our body, including cancer cells.

Without glucose, or at a time when the body is experiencing glucose deficiency, cells are considering ketone bodies to burn fat to survive. However, this does not apply to cancer cells, since they do not have the metabolic flexibility to do so. They will starve and the development process will be slow down. Moreover, they can even die, thereby increasing the real chances of patients recovering. Thus, a ketogenic diet is an additional chance to be cured of cancer.

What to Eat and What to Avoid on Ketogenic Diet?

Here you can find a list of products that you can eat freely and products you need to avoid while being in Keto.

Eat Freely

Animal Sources

- Grass-fed meat (beef, lamb, etc)
- Pastured pork and poultry
- Eggs
- Gelatin
- Ghee
- Butter
- Offal from grass-fed animals

Fats

- Saturated fats
- Monounsaturated
- Polyunsaturated omega-3, especially from animal sources (fatty fish and seafood)

Non-starchy vegetables

- Leafy greens
- Kale
- Kohlrabi
- Radishes
- Celery stalk
- Asparagus
- Cucumber
- Summer squash
- Zucchini
- Bamboo shoots

Fruits

- Avocado

Beverages and Condiments

- Water
- Coffee (black or coconut milk)
- Tea (black, herbal)
- Mayonnaise
- Mustard,
- Pesto,
- Handmade bone broth
- All spices and herbs
- Lemon or lime juice and zest

Eat Sometimes

- Vegetables and Fruits
- Cabbage
- Cauliflower
- broccoli
- Brussels sprouts
- Fennel
- Turnips
- Eggplant
- Tomatoes
- Peppers
- Leek
- Onion
- Garlic
- Mushrooms
- Pumpkin
- Okra
- Bean sprouts
- French artichokes
- Berries (blackberries, blueberries, strawberries, raspberries, cranberries, mulberries, etc.)
- Coconut
- Olives

Animal Sources

- Try to avoid grain-fed animal sources because of high in omega-6

Nuts and seeds

- Pecans
- Almonds
- Walnuts
- Hazelnuts
- Pine nuts
- Flaxseed
- Pumpkin seeds
- Sesame seeds
- Brazil nuts

Condiments

- Stevia
- Sugar-free tomato puree
- Ketchup
- Cocoa powder
- Extra dark chocolate
- Soy lecithin

Alcohol

- Dry wine
- Spirits (unsweetened)

Completely Avoid

- All grains
- Factory-farmed pork and fish
- Processed foods
- Artificial sweeteners

- Refined fats & oils
- Trans fats such as margarine.
- Milk (only small amounts of raw, full-fat milk is allowed)
- Alcoholic sweet drinks
- Tropical fruits

Cooking Conversion Chart

Liquid Measures

1 gal = 4 qt = 8 pt = 16 cups = 128 fl oz
½ gal = 2 qt = 4 pt = 8 cups = 64 fl oz
¼ gal = 1 qt = 2 pt = 4 cups = 32 fl oz
½ qt = 1 pt = 2 cups = 16 fl oz
¼ qt = ½ pt = 1 cup = 8 fl oz

Dry Measures

1 cup = 16 Tbsp = 48 tsp = 250ml
¾ cup = 12 Tbsp = 36 tsp = 175ml
⅔ cup = 10 ⅔ Tbsp = 32 tsp = 150ml
½ cup = 8 Tbsp = 24 tsp = 125ml
⅓ cup = 5 ⅓ Tbsp = 16 tsp = 75ml
¼ cup = 4 Tbsp = 12 tsp = 50ml
⅛ cup = 2 Tbsp = 6 tsp = 30ml
1 Tbsp = 3 tsp = 15ml

Dash or Pinch or Speck = less than ⅛ tsp

Quickies

1 fl oz = 30 ml
1 oz = 28.35 g
1 lb = 16 oz (454 g)
1 kg = 2.2 lb
1 quart = 2 pints

U.S.   Canadian

¼ tsp   1.25 mL
½ tsp   2.5 mL
1 tsp   5 mL
1 Tbl   15 mL
¼ cup   50 mL
⅓ cup   75 mL
½ cup   125 mL
⅔ cup   150 mL
¾ cup   175 mL
1 cup   250 mL
1 quart 1 liter

Recipe Abbreviations

Cup = c or C
Fluid = fl
Gallon = gal
Ounce = oz
Package = pkg
Pint = pt
Pound = lb or #
Quart = qt
Square = sq
Tablespoon = T or Tbl
  or TBSP or TBS
Teaspoon = t or tsp

*Some measurements were rounded

Fahrenheit (°F) to Celcius (°C)

°C = (°F - 32) x 5/9

°F	°C
32°F	0°C
40°F	4°C
140°F	60°C
150°F	65°C
160°F	70°C
225°F	107°C
250°F	121°C
275°F	135°C
300°F	150°C
325°F	165°C
350°F	177°C
375°F	190°C
400°F	205°C
425°F	220°C
450°F	230°C
475°F	245°C
500°F	260°C

OVEN TEMPERATURES

WARMING: 200°F
VERY SLOW: 250°F - 275°F
SLOW: 300°F - 325°F
MODERATE: 350°F - 375°F
HOT: 400°F - 425°F
VERY HOT: 450°F - 475°F

8 Weight Loss Tips

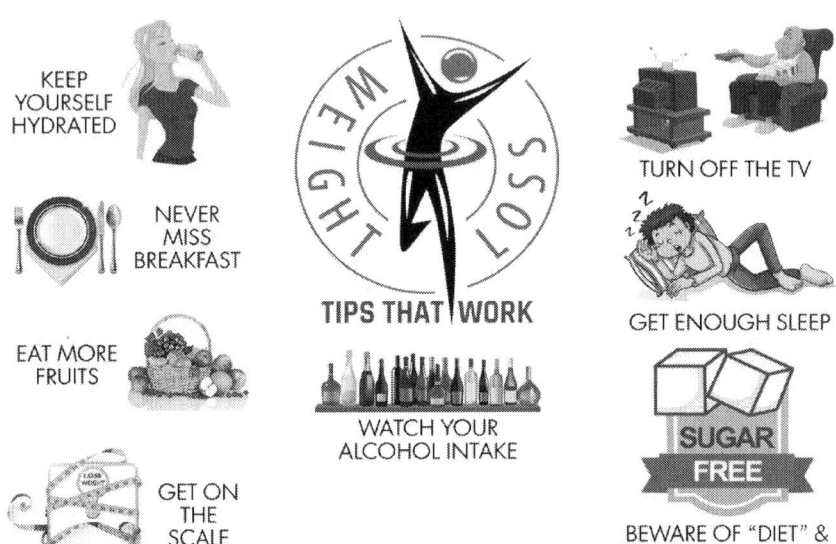

Breakfast Recipes

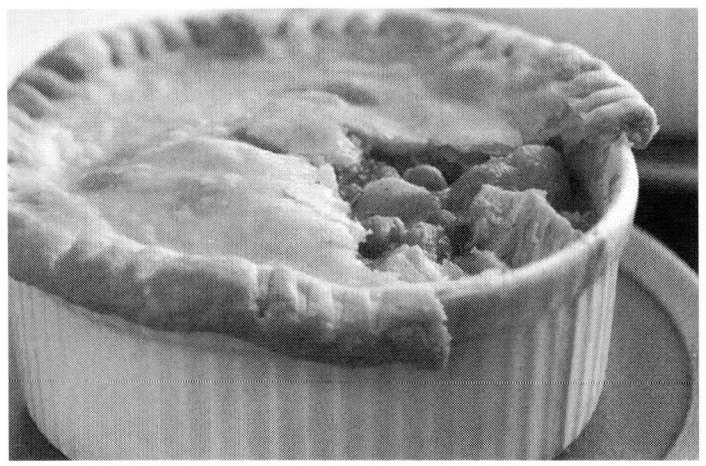

Recipe 1: Crusted Turkey Pots

Ingredients

Crust:
- Almond flour 4 oz.
- Coconut flour 2 oz.
- Baking powder 2 tsp.
- Himalaya salt ¼ tsp.
- Dried dill ¼ tsp.
- Large egg 1
- Mozzarella cheese 12 oz.
- Ghee 6 oz.

Filling:
- Turkey breast 1 lb.
- Ghee 2 tbsp.
- Red onions 1 oz.
- Celery stalks 2
- Carrot 1 oz.

- Sage leaves ¼ tsp.
- Vinegar 1 tbsp.
- Heavy cream 4 oz.
- Peas 1 oz.
- Paprika 2 tsp.
- Salt and pepper to taste

Preparation Method

1. At first, preheat your oven to 350F then grease your muffin or cupcakes with ghee.
2. Now, we can make filling by placing pan over medium heat and add ghee. When ghee is hot add diced turkey and cook until it roasted.
3. Add remaining all ingredients and cook for 15 minutes then keep aside.
4. Now you can start making crust, by mixing all crust ingredients one by one in log shape. It should be soft then divide it into 12 equal parts.
5. Roll each piece and place two rolls on each other than press over muffin tins.
6. Now, fill the muffins cups with cooled filling and top with one more roll.
7. Finally place in preheated oven and cook for 25 minutes or until you find golden brown on top of muffins.
8. Let it cool for 5 minutes and enjoy the taste with your family.

Nutritional Information

- Preparation Time: 45 minutes
- Total servings: 4
- Calories: 454 (per serving)
- Fat: 41.4g
- Protein: 19g
- Carbs: 6.6g

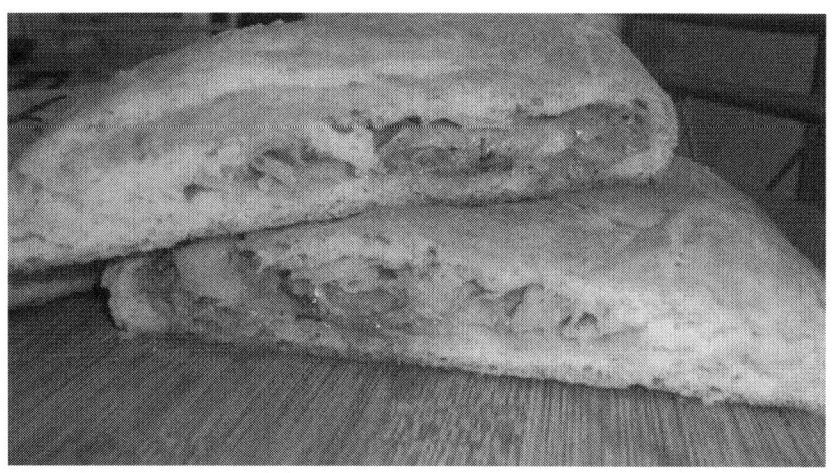

Recipe 2: Cabbage Bread

Ingredients

Bread:
- Chia flour 7 oz.
- Pumpkin spice 2 tsp.
- Cream of tartar 1 tsp.
- Baking soda ¼ tsp.
- Lemons zest 1 tbsp.
- Ghee 2 oz.
- Large eggs 4
- Erythritol 3 oz.
- Cinnamon 1 tsp.
- Cabbages puree 5 oz.

Topping:
- Cream cheese 21 oz.
- Small egg 1
- Erythritol 1.5 oz.
- Cinnamon ½ tsp.
- Cabbages puree 3.5 oz.
- Lemons zest 1 tbsp.
- Pinch of salt

Preparation Method
1. At first, preheat your oven to 300F. In a large bowl, add chia flour, cinnamon, pumpkin spice, cream of tartar, baking soda and mix well and add eggs, ghee, Erythritol, cinnamon and mix well.
2. Add a spoon of cabbages puree and mix well (fresh puree gives better taste then canned).
3. Now, add juice and zest half of a lemon and mix. In another bowl, prepare the cheesecake topping by mixing all topping ingredients.
4. Spoon the bread batter into a baking dish suitable for bread and distribute evenly using a ladle. Add a layer using half of the cheese mixture on top of the bread batter and spread evenly.
5. Mix the remaining cheese mixture with the cabbages puree. Gently spoon the cabbage cheese mixture on top and spread evenly. Transfer into the preheated oven and bake for 60 minutes, make sure that bread is not going to burnt on top.
6. Carefully remove from the baking dish, slice into 12 pieces and enjoy the taste.

Nutritional Information
- Preparation Time: 80 minutes
- Total servings: 12
- Calories: 309 (per serving)
- Fat: 30.3g
- Protein: 9.9g
- Carbs: 5.4g

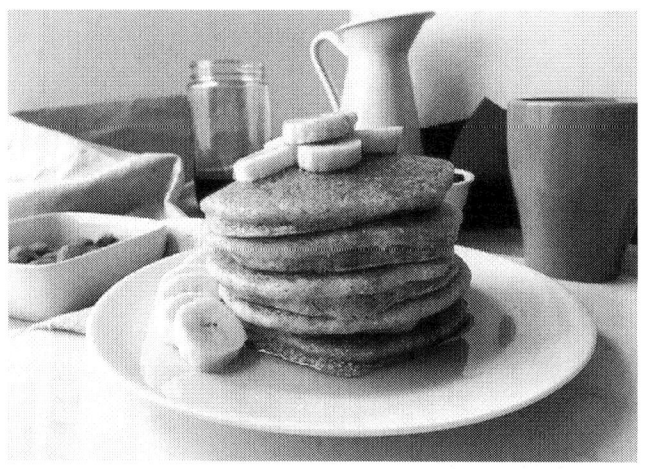

Recipe 3: Flax Pancakes

Ingredients

- Flax meal 1 cup
- Large eggs 2
- Maple syrup 1 tbsp.
- Cabbage puree 2 fl oz
- Cream ¼ cup
- Ghee 2 tbsp.
- All spice 1 tsp.
- Baking soda ½ tsp.
- Salt to taste

Preparation Method

1. Mix eggs, cabbage puree, maple, cream and ghee together without lumps.
2. Mix flax meal, all spice, baking soda and salt together in separate bowl.
3. Slowly start adding wet mixture (step1) to get smooth consistency by adding butter.
4. Heat the pan and grease the pan with butter, then add the pancake batter into the pan and cook until bubbles appears on the top.

5. Flip it and cook other side until browned and serve when it is warm for a nice taste.

Nutritional Information

- Preparation Time: 15 minutes
- Total servings: 8
- Calories: 199.5 (per serving)
- Fat: 16.6g
- Protein: 8.1g
- Carbs: 4g

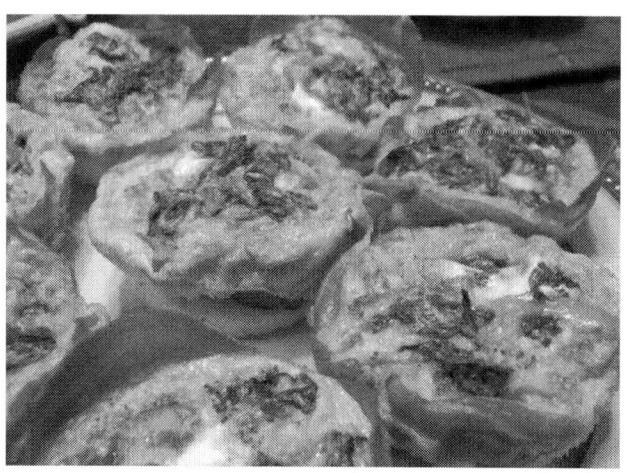

Recipe 4: Crumbled Turnip Eggs Cups

Ingredients

- Ghee 2 tsp.
- Diced shallots 1 oz.
- Turnips greens 3 cups
- Large eggs 4
- Butter 4 tsp.
- Salt and ground pepper to taste
- Blue cheese 1 oz.
- Mascarpone cheese 2 oz.
- Garlic cloves 3
- Grated coconut 1 oz.

Preparation Method

1. Preheat oven to 400F. Easily rinse ramekins with butter. Heat a large pan over medium heat, add ghee, shallots and cook 2 minutes.
2. Add turnips, salt and pepper and boil until the spinach fades for about 3 minutes. Mix in blue cheese, mascarpone and remove from the heat.
3. Divide the faded kale under the oven-proof food and make a fountain in the middle of each. Beat egg into

each dish and season with grated coconut, cloves, salt and pepper.
4. Place on the baking sheets and bake until the white is set and the yolks are tight around the edges, but still soft in the middle, about 15 minutes and serve immediately.

Nutritional Information

- Preparation Time: 25 minutes
- Total servings: 4
- Calories: 240 (per serving)
- Fat: 20.9g
- Protein: 11.9g
- Carbs: 6.3g

Lunch Recipes

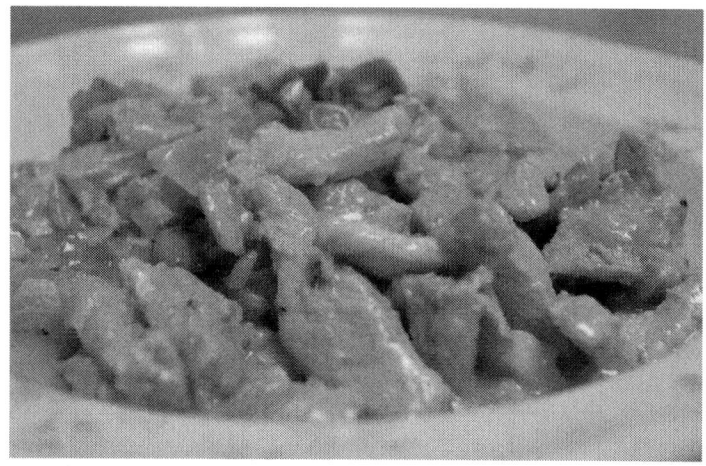

Recipe 5: Coconut Pork Stew

Ingredients

- Pork 1 lb.
- Ghee 1 oz.
- Onion powder 1 tbsp.
- Garlic powder 2 tsp.
- Ginger powder 1 tsp.
- All spice 1 tsp.
- Salt to taste
- Diced tomatoes 2 oz.
- Coconut milk 4 oz.
- Parsley 1 tbsp.

Preparation Method

1. Cut the pork into small cube size pieces and season with salt, pepper and ground pepper, ginger, garlic and mix well.

2. Add tomatoes and mix well. Finally, add coconut milk and mix.
3. Cook for 40 minutes on medium heat and mix thoroughly then sprinkle chopped parsley. Serve over cauliflower rice or normal rice for nice taste.

Nutritional Information
- Preparation Time: 45 minutes
- Total servings: 5
- Calories: 501 (per serving)
- Fat: 40.8g
- Protein: 25.5g
- Carbs:5g

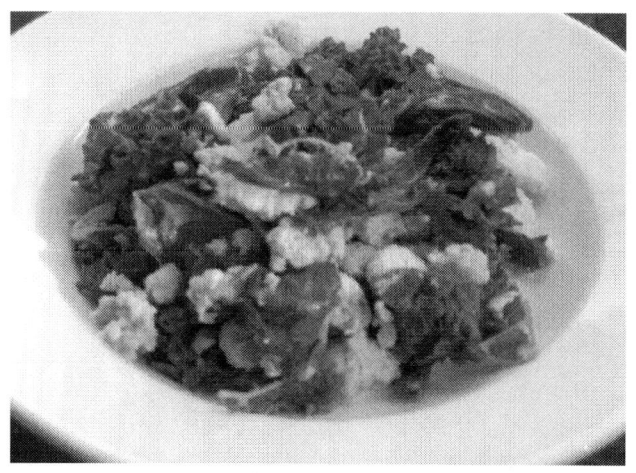

Recipe 6: Coconut Turkey Stew

Ingredients

- Onions 2 oz.
- Garlic powder 1 tsp.
- Ginger powder 1 tsp.
- Ghee 2 tsp.
- Turkey 1 lb.
- Coconut milk 1 cup
- Parsley 1 tbsp.
- Cumin powder 1 tsp.
- Green chili 1 tsp.
- Turmeric 1 tsp.
- Frozen black beans 2 oz.
- Brazil nuts 2 oz.
- Tomato sauce 1 oz.
- Salt and fresh pepper to taste

Preparation Method

1. Heat in a large skillet pan; add ghee and onions on medium heat. Cook about 10 minutes. Add garlic and ginger, cook for another 2 minutes.

2. Add lamb to the pan and brown. Season with salt, pepper, cumin, coriander, green chili, turmeric and mix well.
3. Add coconut milk, brazil nuts, tomato sauce and water. Reduce heat to simmer about 20 minutes. Add frozen peas and simmer for an additional 15 minutes or until desired taste comes.

Nutritional Information
- Preparation Time: 35 minutes
- Total servings: 4
- Calories: 380.3 (per serving)
- Fat: 32.6g
- Protein: 17.2g
- Carbs: 8g

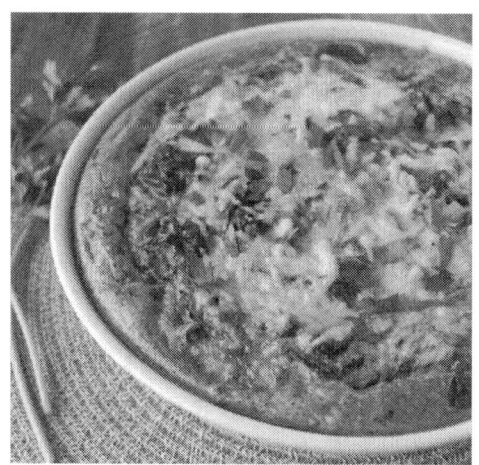

Recipe 7: Turkey Quiche

Ingredients
Crust
- Ground turkey 5 oz.
- Coconut flour 5 oz.
- Chia meal 3 tbsp.
- Large eggs 3
- Salt ½ tsp.

Filling
- Large eggs 6
- Ghee 1 tbsp.
- Heavy whipping cream 4 fl oz.
- Spring onions 1 oz.
- Cheddar cheese 7 oz.
- Mascarpone cheese 4 oz.
- Cream cheese 8 oz.
- Asparagus spears 8 oz.
- Salt and pepper to taste
- Fennel for garnish

Preparation Method
1. At first, preheat the oven to 400F. Put ground turkey into a food processor or blender and make powder.

2. Add powdered rind in a mixing bowl together with the coconut flour and chia meal, Himalaya salt and mix until well combined.
3. Now, crack the eggs and mix the dough using hand or hand mixer, place this dough in a rectangular baking tray with removable bottom (30 x 20 cm / 12 x 8 inch).
4. Bake in preheated oven for 15 minutes and keep aside until it cools down. Reduce the oven to 350F.
5. Now, add shredded cheese's (cheddar and mascarpone) over cooled crust and keep aside. Meantime, take a large bowl and crack the eggs, add the cream, season with salt and pepper and whisk until it combines well
6. On the other hand, place a pan over medium heat with ghee. When ghee is hot, add sliced spring onions and cook for 3 minutes or until fragrant. Add this to the egg mixture and combine well. Add cream cheese to egg mixture and pour over shredded cheese.
7. Now, top egg mixture with asparagus and place in preheated oven for 30 minutes or until lightly browned and crispy on top.
8. Garnish with freshly chopped fennel and enjoy the taste.

Nutritional Information

- Preparation Time: 60 minutes
- Total servings: 8
- Calories: 600 (per serving)
- Fat: 44.1g
- Protein: 24.4g
- Carbs: 6.5g

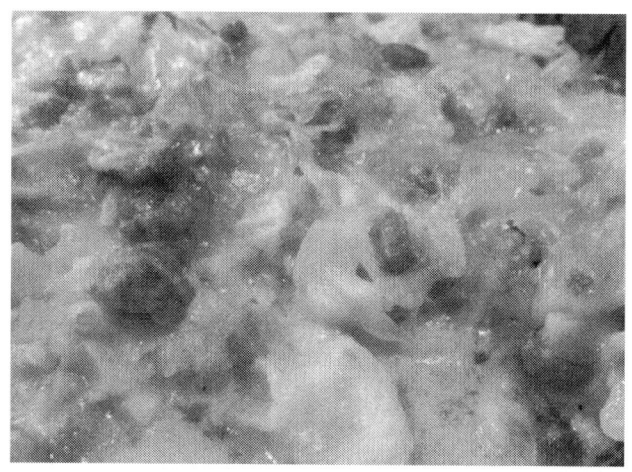

Recipe 8: Cabbage Cheese Meal

Ingredients
- Ghee 1 tbsp.
- Egg 1
- Cream cheese 1 tbsp.
- Mozzarella 1 tbsp.
- Mascarpone cheese 1tbsp.
- Flax flour 2 tbsp.
- Chia meal 1 tbsp.
- Baking soda ½ tsp.
- Salt to taste

Filling
- Cabbage 2 oz.
- Bacon slices 2
- Roasted garlic cloves 3

Toppings
- Mayonnaise 2 tbsp.
- Vinegar 1 tsp.
- BBQ sauce 1 tbsp.
- Sage 1 tbsp.

Preparation Method

1. In a small bowl mix mayonnaise, rice vinegar and keep aside. In a mixing bowl, add ghee, cream cheese, mascarpone, mozzarella and mix until softened.
2. Now, add almond flour, chia meal, baking soda, salt to the mixing bowl and mix well. Now, add egg into the batter, add cabbage and stir until fully incorporated.
3. Place large skillet over medium heat and add sliced bacon until it becomes crispy.
4. Spread incorporated batter into bacon skillet and cook for 5 minutes or until batter turns to golden color on the bottom.
5. Flip and cook again 5 minutes and transfer to a plate. Spread BBQ sauce, mayonnaise, vinegar and roasted garlic.
6. Finally, sprinkle sage and enjoy the taste.

Nutritional Information

- Preparation Time: 30 minutes
- Total servings: 2
- Calories: 498 (per serving)
- Fat: 46.2g
- Protein: 12.5g
- Carbs: 5.2g

Dinner Recipes

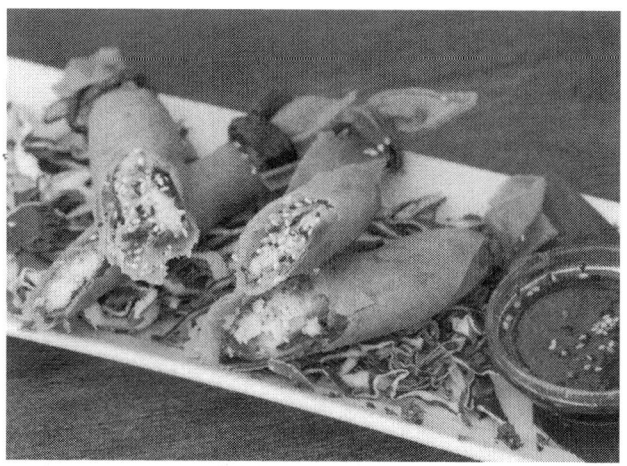

Recipe 9: Mascarpone Salmon Wraps

Ingredients

- Large eggs 3
- Avocado 3.5 oz.
- Smoked salmon 2 oz.
- Mascarpone cheese 2 tbsp.
- Fresh dill 2 tbsp.
- Cabbage 4 tbsp.
- Ghee 1 tbsp.
- Salt and pepper to taste

Preparation Method

1. At first, whisk egg, salt and pepper in a small bowl, add mascarpone cheese with chopped dill and keep aside.
2. Place pan over medium heat and add ghee, cabbage. When ghee is hot, add egg mixture into pan and cook for 1 minute each side.

3. Meanwhile, slice the smoked salmon, avocado and keep aside. Now, place the omelet on a plate and add sliced salmon, avocado and fold into a wrap.

Nutritional Information
- Preparation Time: 15 minutes
- Total servings: 2
- Calories: 388.7 (per serving)
- Fat: 34.6g
- Protein: 16.6g
- Carbs: 4.2g

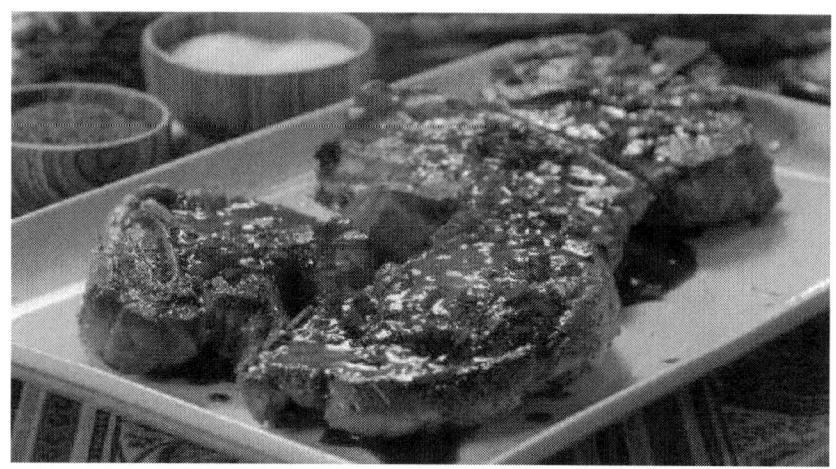

Recipe 10: Vinaigrette Lamb Fry

Ingredients

Lamb Chops
- Lamb chops 4
- Ghee 1 oz.
- Salt and pepper to taste
- Paprika 1 tsp.
- Small better melon 1
- Catnip 1 tsp.

Vinaigrette
- Vinegar 2 tbsp.
- Lemon juice 1 tbsp.
- Maple syrup 1 tbsp.
- Salt and pepper to taste

Topping
- Parsley 1 tbsp.

Preparation Method

1. At first, season lamb chops with salt, pepper, ghee and keep aside.
2. Place large iron skillet over high heat and add seasoned lamb chops and cook 10 minutes both side.

3. Decrease the heat to medium and add better melon slices, catnip over the lamb chops and place in the oven for about 10 minutes at 350F.
4. Meanwhile, prepare vinaigrette by mixing all the ingredients together. When lamb chops are ready, pour vinaigrette over top then sprinkle parsley and serve hot.

Nutritional Information
- Preparation Time: 25 minutes
- Total servings: 2
- Calories: 488 (per serving)
- Fat: 40.7g
- Protein: 21.3g
- Carbs: 5.3g

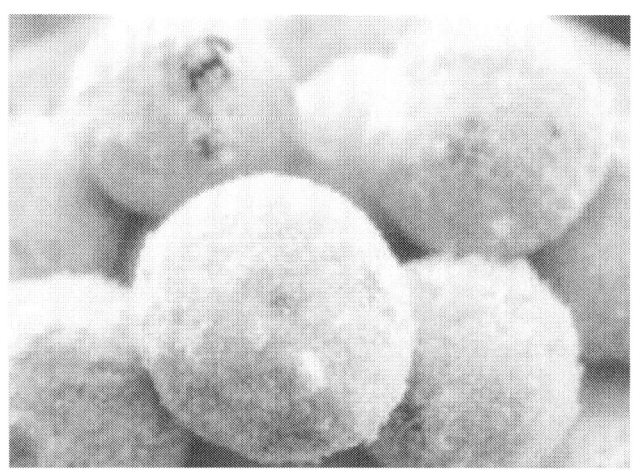

Recipe 11: Ghee Rind Balls

Ingredients

Meatballs
- Ghee 1 tbsp.
- Ground rind 0.5 lb.
- Onions 1 oz.
- Garlic cloves 2
- Flax meal 1 oz.
- Coconut milk 1 tbsp.
- Salt to taste

Coconut Broth
- Coconut milk 2 oz.
- Broth 2 oz.

Spices
- Coriander seeds 1 tsp.
- Turmeric ½ tsp.
- Cinnamon ½ tsp.
- Red pepper ½ tsp.
- Ginger powder ½ tsp.
- Garlic powder ½ tsp.
- Chili paste 1 tsp.

Preparation Method
1. In a large pan, add ghee. When ghee is hot, add garlic, onions and cook until fragrant and translucent.
2. Meantime, combine flax meal, coconut milk, ground rind, salt and create a paste.
3. Add onions, garlic to this paste and create small balls using hand. Place the pan over medium heat and add ghee. When ghee is hot add meatballs all over the pan (ca. 15 minutes).
4. When meat are browned on both sides, add coconut milk, broth, and all spices, mix well and cook for 20 more minutes.
5. Finally, serve with some coconut broth with meatballs in a bowl and enjoy the taste.

Nutritional Information
- Preparation Time: 30 minutes
- Total servings: 2
- Calories: 572 (per serving)
- Fat: 46.9g
- Protein: 23.4g
- Carbs: 5.4g

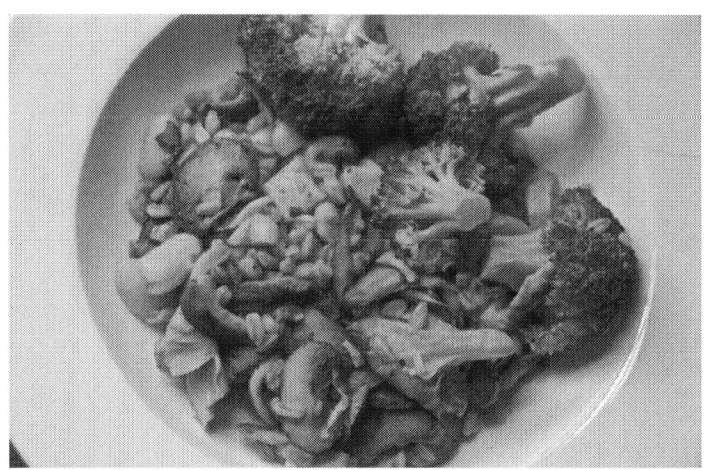

Recipe 12: Forest Mushroom Broccoli Bowl

Ingredients

- Macadamia nuts ½ cup
- Coriander 2 cups
- Ginger paste 2 tsp.
- Lemon juice 2 tbsp.
- Salt and pepper to taste
- Mascarpone cheese 3 oz.
- Forest mushrooms 1 lb.
- Broccoli 2 oz.
- Ghee 1 tbsp.

Preparation Method

1. At first, soak macadamia nuts overnight in water then drain water and add macadamia nuts, coriander, ginger, lemon juice, salt, and pepper to food processor then process until smooth.
2. Now, cook broccoli in small pan over medium heat for 10 minutes and keep aside then place large skillet over medium heat with ghee and add forest mushrooms, season with salt and pepper then cook for 10 minutes, don't forget to stir occasionally until all the water has evaporated and they begin to brown and keep aside.

3. Finally, add broccoli, a quarter of the forest mushrooms, mascarpone and top with a tablespoon of the pesto in bowl and enjoy the delicious taste.

Nutritional Information
- Preparation Time: 35 minutes
- Total servings: 4
- Calories: 381 (per serving)
- Fat: 34.4g
- Protein: 15.3g
- Carbs:7g

Soup Recipes

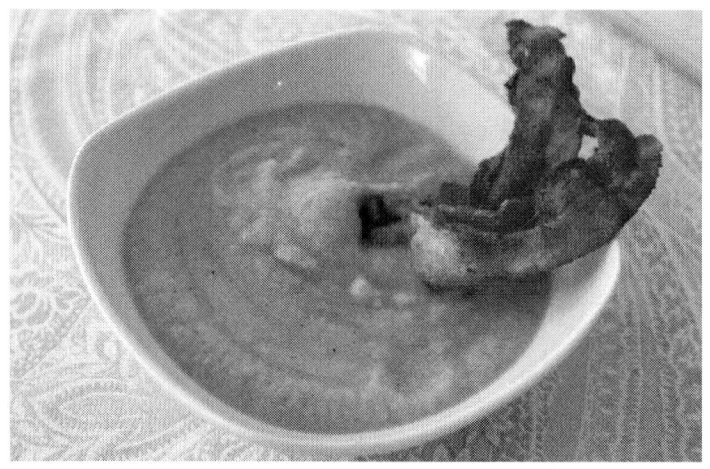

Recipe 13: Bacon Broccoli Soup

Ingredients
- Vegetable broth 1 ½ cups
- Bacon 4 slices
- Broccoli puree 1 cup
- Ghee 1 oz.
- Butter 1 oz.
- Garlic 1 tsp.
- Ginger 1 tsp.
- Salt ½ tsp.
- Pepper ½ tsp.
- Red chili flakes 2
- Fresh ginger ½ tsp.
- Mint ¼ tsp.
- Bay leaf 1
- Mascarpone cheese 1 oz.

Preparation Method
1. Keep saucepan over medium heat, add ghee. When ghee is hot, add garlic and fresh ginger.
2. Let this sauté for about 3 minutes or until onions start to go translucent then add spices (salt, pepper, coriander, bay leaf, red chili flakes) to the pan and let cook for 2 minutes. Add broccoli puree to pan and stir into the onions and spices well
3. Once the broccoli is mixed well, add vegetable broth to the pan. Stir until everything is combined.
4. Bring to a boil to simmer for 20 minutes. Once simmered, use an immersion blender to blend together all of the ingredients. You want a smooth puree here so make sure you take your time. Cook for an additional 20 minutes.
5. In the meantime, cook 4 slices of bacon over medium heat. Once the soup is ready, pour mascarpone cheese and the grease from the cooked bacon and mix well.
1. Crumble the bacon over the top of the soup and enjoy the taste of the soup.

Nutritional Information
- Preparation Time: 45 minutes
- Serving per Recipe: 3
- Calories:491 (per serving)
- Fat: 45.1g
- Protein: 10.8g
- Carbs: 5.7g

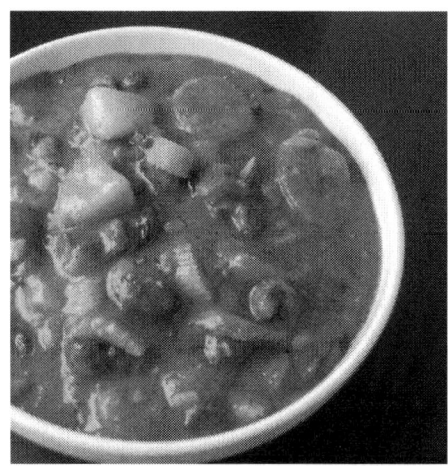

Recipe 14: Soy Lamb Soup

Ingredients
- Lamb bone 1 lb.
- Onion Powder 1 tsp.
- Garlic Powder 1 tsp.
- Ginger powder 1 tsp.
- Chili powder ½ tsp.
- Ghee 2 oz.
- Soy sauce 2 oz.
- Broth 3 cups
- Cream cheese 2 oz.
- Cumin powder 1 tsp.
- Salt and Pepper to taste

Preparation Method
2. Cut or slice the lamb bones into chunks and drop them in the pot and add all the rest of the ingredients to the cooking pot except cream, cheese.
3. Set cooking pot on heat for 60 minutes and cooks completely. Once everything is cooked, remove the lamb from the cooking pot and shred using a fork.
4. Add cream and cheese to the cooking pot. Using an immersion blender, emulsify all of the liquids together.

This will help the soup from separating while you are eating.
5. Place the lamb back into the cooking pot, stir together. Taste and season with extra salt, pepper, cumin and soy sauce. Serve and enjoy the taste.

Nutritional Information

- Preparation Time: 190 minutes
- Serving per Recipe: 5
- Calories:531.2 (per serving)
- Fat: 46.3g
- Protein: 22.1g
- Carbs: 5.4g

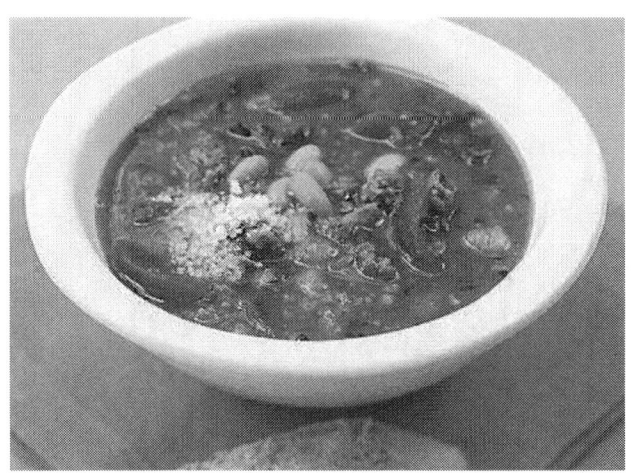

Recipe 15: Lamb Sausage Soup

Ingredients

- Ground lamb 1 lb.
- Sausage 7 oz.
- Fresh tomatoes 7 oz.
- Tomato Puree 2 oz.
- Onions 2 oz.
- Garlic 3 cloves
- Ginger powder ½ tsp.
- Ghee 4 tbsp.
- Salt and pepper to taste
- Broth 1 liter
- Garnish with sweet marjoram

Preparation Method

1. At first, dice the onion, sausage, tomatoes and keep aside.
2. Place large Dutch pan over medium heat with ghee. Once ghee hot, add the diced onion, garlic, ginger and cook 2 minutes or until lightly browned, cook for 5 minutes, don't forget to stir to prevent burning.

3. Add the sausage, ground lamb into the pot and cook until it turns to brown color. Add the chopped tomatoes, tomato puree.
4. Now, add broth (your choice) and season with salt and pepper. Cook the soup until bubbles appears and before serving, add chopped sweet marjoram for extra flavor.

Nutritional Information
- Preparation Time: 30 minutes
- Total servings: 5
- Calories: 371 (per serving)
- Fat: 32g
- Protein: 15.3g
- Carbs: 6.1g

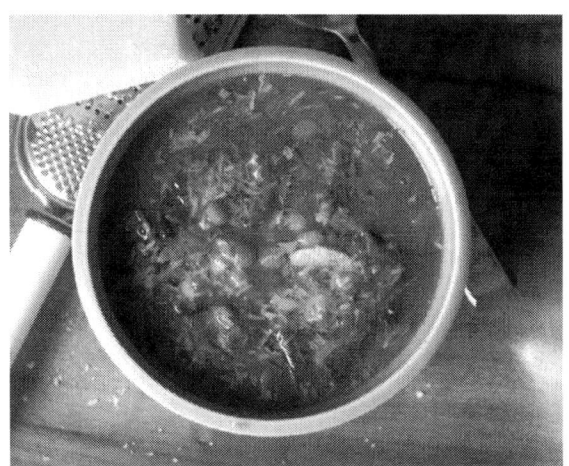

Recipe 16: Red Chard Cheese Soup

Ingredients

- Ghee 1 tbsp.
- Onion 1 oz.
- Red chard 10 oz.
- Large eggs 8
- Goat cheese 8 oz.
- Mascarpone cheese 2 oz.
- Sea salt 1 tsp.
- Black pepper ½ tsp.

Preparation Method

1. At first, preheat your oven to 350F and place your pan over medium heat. When ghee is hot, add onions and cook until it becomes soft.
2. Add chopped chard and cook for 2 minutes and keep aside. In a bowl, mix egg, goat cheese, mascarpone, salt, pepper and add to mixture.
3. Using blender, blend the mixture and pour into pan, place in preheated oven for 30 minutes and enjoy the taste.

Nutritional Information

- Preparation Time: 40 minutes
- Total servings: 4
- Calories: 580 (per serving)
- Fat: 48g
- Protein: 27.1g
- Carbs: 6.9g

Salad Recipes

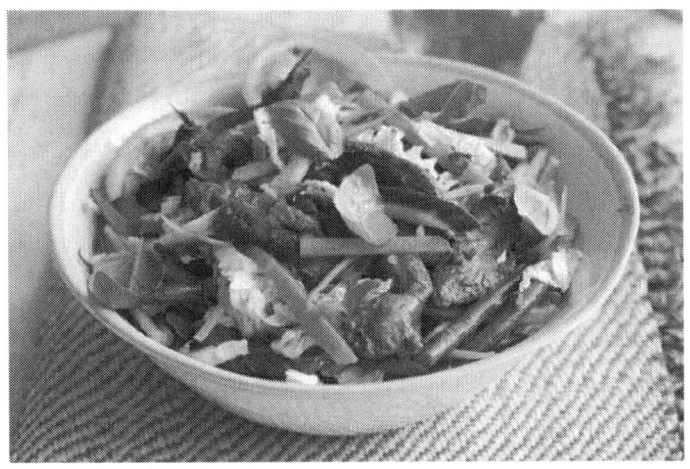

Recipe 17: Sweet Cheese Duck Salad

Ingredients
- Duck breasts 14 oz.
- Bacon slices 4 oz.
- Dates 2 (chopped)
- Romaine lettuce 1.76 lb.
- Salad Dressing 8 tbsp.
- Mascarpone cheese 4 oz.
- Salt and pepper to taste
- Anchovies 1 oz.

Preparation Method
1. At first, preheat your oven to 375F and bake bacons until it becomes crispy approximately 15 minutes and keep aside.
2. Now, make duck breast fry, by placing in oven to 430F, don't forget to season with salt and pepper. Cook for 15 minutes or until golden color and keep aside.

3. Meanwhile, prepare dressing and other ingredients. Use a peeler to make the mascarpone flakes, dates and place the lettuce in a serving bowl and toss with the dressing.
4. Now, slice the duck breasts into thin strips and place on top of the lettuce. Add the mascarpone flakes and crisped up and crumbled bacon, anchovies and enjoy the taste.

Nutritional Information
- Preparation Time: 45 minutes
- Total servings: 4
- Calories: 656 (per serving)
- Fat: 52.5g
- Protein: 28.6g
- Carbs: 7.1g

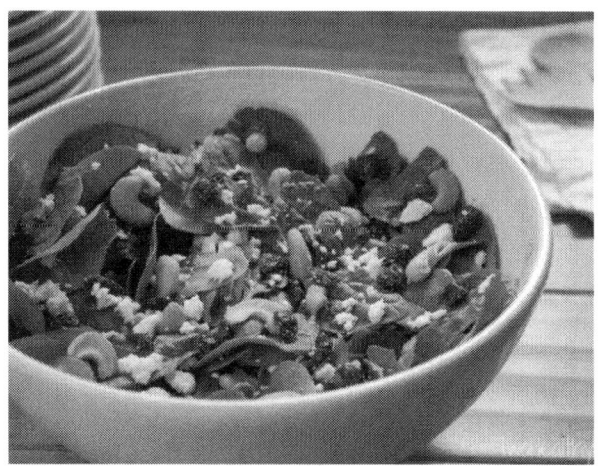

Recipe 18: Green Nut Salad

Ingredients
- Mixed greens 1 oz. (spinach, rapini, collards)
- Fresh herbs 1 oz. (Mint, Marjoram)
- Roasted pine nuts 1 oz.
- Pistachio 2 tbsp.
- Vinaigrette 1 ½ tbsp.
- Parmesan cheese 1 tbsp.
- Mascarpone cheese 1 tbsp.
- Bacon slices 2
- Ghee 1 tbsp.
- Salt and pepper to taste

Preparation Method
1. Cook bacon until crisp. Measure your greens, herbs and set in a container that can be shaken.
2. Crumble bacon, then add the rest of the ingredients to the greens and shake the container with a lid.
3. Add your seasonings and ghee for better taste and shake once again for proper dressing. Serve and enjoy the taste.

Nutritional Information

- Preparation Time: 10 minutes
- Total servings: 2
- Calories: 341 (per serving)
- Fat: 28.3g
- Protein: 11.2g
- Carbs: 5.2g

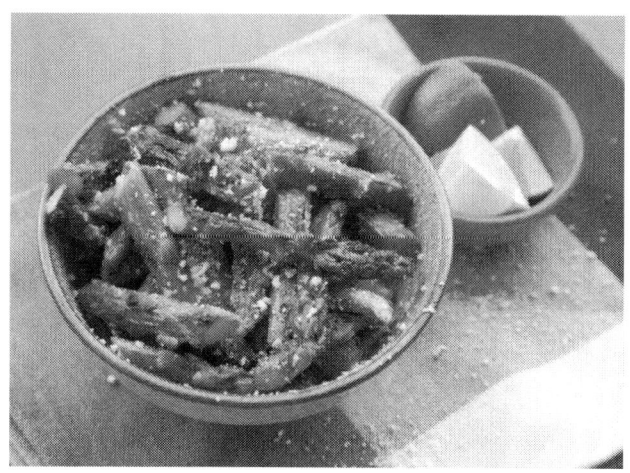

Recipe 19: Cheesy Asparagus Salad

Ingredients
- Asparagus 2 oz. (cooked)
- Pine nuts 1 oz. (roasted)
- Vinaigrette 4 tsp.
- Parmesan cheese 1 tbsp.
- Mascarpone cheese 1 oz.
- Bacon 2 slices
- Salt and pepper to taste

Preparation Method
1. Cook bacon until crisp. Measure your asparagus and set in a container that can be shaken.
2. Crumble bacon, then add the rest of the ingredients to the beans and shake the container with a lid.
3. Add your seasonings for better taste and shake once again for proper dressing.
4. Before serving, add mozzarella balls and enjoy the taste.

Nutritional Information
- Preparation Time: 10 minutes

- Serving per Recipe: 1
- Calories: 534 (per serving)
- Fat: 40.7g
- Protein: 18.1g
- Carbs: 6.2g

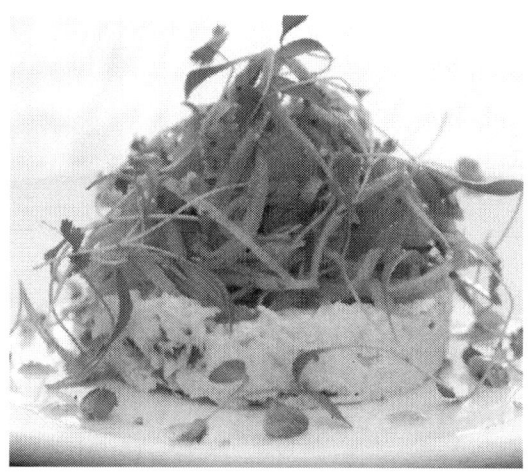

Recipe 20: Crab Carrot Salad

Ingredients

- Carrot 1 cup
- Crab meat 4 oz.
- Lemon juice 1 tbsp.
- Grape tomatoes 4
- Mascarpone 1 oz.
- Ghee 1 oz.
- Salt and pepper to taste
- Butter salad leaves 2
- Macadamia nuts 1 oz.

Preparation Method

1. In a medium bowl, add lemon juice, tomato, ghee, salt and fresh pepper. Add crab meat and sway lightly.
2. Cut the carrot and season with the remaining ingredients, mix carrot, crab and sprinkle smashed macadamia nuts. Serve immediately with butter leaves to enjoy the taste.

Nutritional Information

- Preparation Time: 15 minutes
- Total servings: 2

- Calories: 206 (per serving)
- Fat: 27g
- Protein: 13.2g
- Carbs: 6.6g

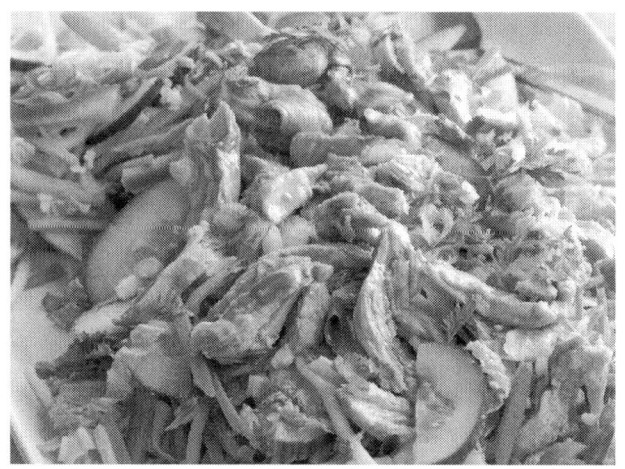

Recipe 21: Turkey Salad

Ingredients

- Spinach 2 oz.
- Dandelion greens ½ oz.
- Roasted Brazil nuts 1 oz.
- Vinaigrette 4 tsp.
- Grated cheese 1 tbsp.
- Mozzarella cheese 1 oz.
- Turkey slices 2 (each 1 oz.)
- Salt and pepper to taste

Preparation Method

1. Cook turkey until crisp. Measure your greens and set in a container that can be shaken.
2. Crumble bacon, then add the rest of the ingredients to the greens and shake the container with a lid.
3. Add your seasonings for better taste and shake once again for proper dressing.
4. Before serving, add mozzarella balls and enjoy the taste.

Nutritional Information

- Preparation Time: 10 minutes
- Serving per Recipe: 1
- Calories: 553 (per serving)
- Fat: 36.4g
- Protein: 16.6g
- Carbs: 7g

Snack Recipes

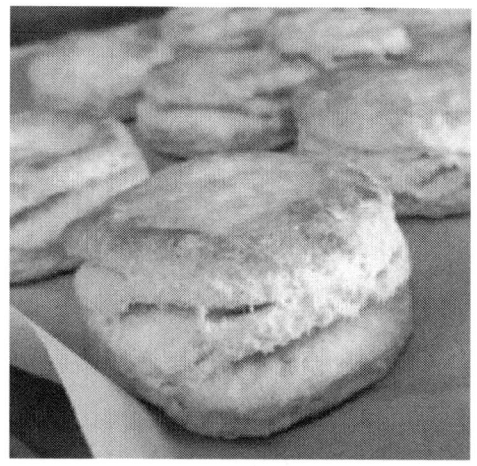

Recipe 22: Cabbage Biscuits

Ingredients

- Almond flour 1 ½ cup
- Cabbage 1.5 lb.
- Cheddar cheese 5 oz.
- Mascarpone cheese 4 oz.
- Ghee 2 oz.
- Large eggs 2
- Salt to taste
- Ginger powder 1 tsp.
- Baking soda ½ tsp.
- Chopped walnuts 2 tbsp.

Preparation Method

1. At first, preheat your oven to 375F, blend cabbage until it is finely chopped.

2. In a large bowl, mix almond flour, salt, peppers, ginger powder, baking soda. Mix it well, add eggs and ghee. Mix until a dough forms.
3. Add your cabbage to the mixture. Combine everything with your hands. Grate cheddar and mascarpone to the dough. Mix everything with the hands until the cheese is evenly distributed.
4. Place your non-stick silpat on a cookie sheet, so that they do not stick as they boil. Form pies from the dough and sprinkle chopped walnuts. Bake like biscuits for 15 minutes or until they begin to flatten.
5. Turn it and continue baking for about 5 minutes then, turn your oven to roast and brew the biscuits for 3 minutes. Let it cool for 2 minutes before you enjoy the taste.

Nutritional Information

- Preparation Time: 30 minutes
- Total servings: 12
- Calories: 189 (per serving)
- Fat: 17.8g
- Protein: 7g
- Carbs: 3.1g

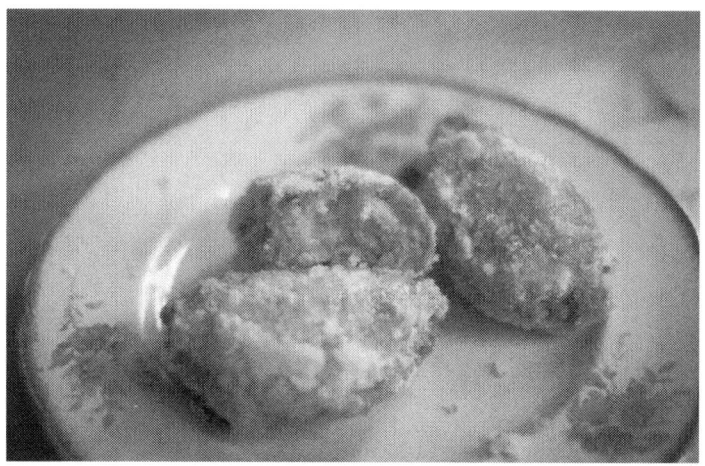

Recipe 23: Banana Bombs

Ingredients

- Ghee 4 oz.
- Heavy whipped cream 4 oz.
- Fresh cheese 4 oz.
- Vanillas extract 1 tsp.
- Stevia 10 drops
- Banana protein powder 1 oz.

Preparation Method

- At first, mix ghee, heavy cream and fresh cheese. Using a mixer, mix all the ingredients together or place in microwave oven for 30 seconds to 1 minute to soften them.
- Add berry extract and liquid stevia to the mixture and mix with a spoon.
- Distribute the mixture into a silicone tray and freeze for 3 hours.

Nutritional Information

- Preparation Time: 182 minutes
- Total servings: 10

- Calories: 186 (per serving)
- Fat: 18g
- Protein: 7.9g
- Carbs: 1g

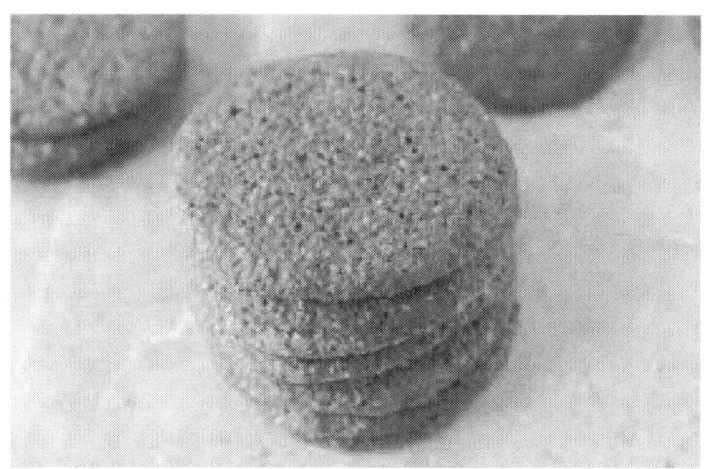

Recipe 24: Crunchy Chia Biscuits

Ingredients
- Chia flour 1 ½ cup
- Ghee 2 oz.
- Salt to taste
- Baking soda ½ tsp.
- Cayenne pepper ¼ tsp.
- Garlic powder 1 tsp.
- Ginger powder 1 tsp.
- Thyme 2 tbsp.

Preparation Method
1. At first, preheat oven to 325F. Place a cookie sheet with parchment paper.
2. In a medium bowl, mix chia flour, pepper, salt and baking powder.
3. Add thyme, cayenne and garlic, ginger and stir until uniformly combined. Next, add to the pesto and snow bake until the dough forms into coarse crumbs.
4. Put the ghee into the cracker mixture with a fork until the dough forms a ball.
5. Transfer the dough to the prepared cookie sheet and spread the dough thinly until it is about 1 mm thick.

Make sure the thickness is the same, so that the biscuits evenly bake.
6. Place the pan in the pre-heated oven then sprinkle thyme over it and bake for 15 minutes to light golden brown color. After baking, remove from the oven and cut into biscuits of the desired size.

Nutritional Information

- Preparation Time: 25 minutes
- Total servings: 6
- Calories:226 (per serving)
- Fat: 21g
- Protein: 5.3g
- Carbs: 2.5g

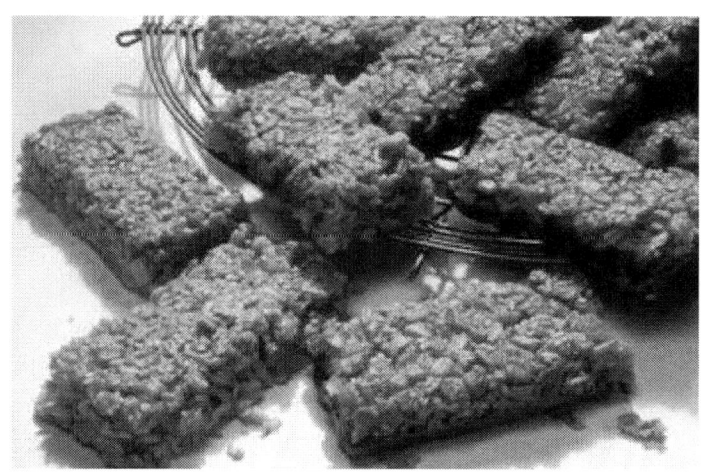

Recipe 25: Protein Flax Bars

Ingredients

- Flax ½ cup
- Ghee 2 oz.
- Maple syrup 1 oz.
- Cinnamon powder 1 tsp.
- Pinch of salt
- Cashew nuts 2 oz.
- Cashew butter 1 oz.
- Protein powder 2 oz.
- Shredded coconut 1 tbsp.

Preparation Method

1. At first, combine flax and melted ghee in a large bowl. Add cinnamon, salt and maple syrup, cashew butter, protein powder and mix well.
2. Add chopped cashews and mix everything evenly. Pour parchment paper into a casserole dish and spread the dough in a flat layer. Sprinkle crushed coconut and cinnamon up for beautiful crispy flavor.
3. Place them in a refrigerator and cool for 3 hours (night will give the best result). Cut into bars and enjoy the taste.

Nutritional Information

- Preparation Time:15 minutes
- Total servings: 8
- Calories: 199.5 (per serving)
- Fat: 21.7g
- Protein: 9.3g
- Carbs: 4.6g

Conclusion

Thank you again for downloading my cookbook! I Hope this book helps you to know more interesting and tasty recipes or inspire you to create your own unique dishes.

Note from the author:

If you've enjoyed this book, I'd greatly appreciate if you could leave an honest review on Amazon. Reviews are very important to us authors, and it only takes a minute for to post.

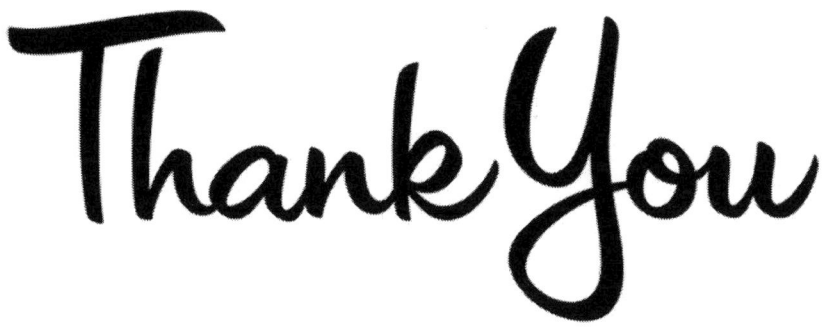

Printed in Germany
by Amazon Distribution
GmbH, Leipzig